25 Herbal Tea's For Optimum Health

By Fly Ty Unchained

Foreword

I was beginning to suffer from aches, pains and certain diseases of the body like acid reflux, and in my opinion, it was mostly due to my lifestyle and diet. As I began to change my eating habits over the years, such as cutting red meat, pork and soda out of my diet, and consuming more water, vegetables and Tea, I began to notice how much better my body felt over all. While I still suffer with mild acid reflux at times, due to my diet change I don't experience nearly as much heartburn and discomfort as I once did. Drinking a cup of Green Tea every morning and then before bed made a big difference in my life and overall health. I hope the information you may find in this book can help you continue to maintain a healthy lifestyle, or maybe start you out on a path to finding Optimum Health…

Peace

Acknowledgements

I would like to thank everyone over the years that pushed me towards living a much healthier lifestyle. Where I come from in the Bronx N.Y. there are very few health food stores or places to buy Organic Herbal Teas, so any one on a healthy path such as myself always gets much respect from me. Knowledge is power and health is wealth, I know those are common clichés we use, but I've found them to be profoundly true and words that I live by. Thank you for opening my eyes to the wrong ways I was eating and the unhealthy beverages I was consuming, while guiding me to a life of hopefully longevity, good health and prosperity. A cup of Tea a day keeps the stress away!

Fly Ty Unchained

Table of Contents:

Introduction ....Page 11

Alfalfa...................Page 13

Basil.....................Page 14

Black Tea..............Page 15

Blessed Thistle.......Page 16

Burdock Root........Page 17

Catnip...................Page 18

Chamomile............Page 19

Chrysanthemum....Page 20

Devil's Claw.........Page 21

Dandelion............Page 22

Echinacea...........Page 23

Dong Quai...........Page 24

Eucalyptus.........Page 25

Fennel................Page 26

Ginger...............Page 25

Gingko Biloba......Page 27

Ginseng.............Page 28

Green Tea...........Page 29

Honeysuckle........Page 30

Hops..................Page 31

Hyssop...............Page 32

Jasmine...............Page 33

Peppermint...........Page 34

Valerian Root........Page 35

Introduction

Tea is considered the most consumed beverage in the world behind water. The further I studied into the world of Tea, the more I was astounded at how beneficial drinking tea on a daily basis can be. Whether you're trying to maintain good health or get back to optimum health, Tea should be one of the major things that you consume at least once a day. From Honeysuckle to Jasmine Tea, when combined with honey and lemon (If you choose) it can make for a healthy refreshing drink. Instead of coffee filled with caffeine or a glass of acid filled soda, try drinking more Tea and see the difference in how you feel. Some of the healthiest people in the world consume Tea on a daily basis, and I highly recommend you make it part of your diet too!

Peace...

Alfalfa

Alfalfa Herb tea can be used as a remedy for many digestive issues and other ailments. Alfalfa tea has been known to aid in the relief of arthritis symptoms

Alfalfa Tea Benefits:

Cleansing the blood, liver and bowel

Encouraging appetite

Promoting weight gain

Kidney problems

Curing Auto-immune disorder

Lowering cholesterol

Preventing strokes

*Alfalfa Tea Warnings:

For most people, Alfalfa is safe, but it may interact with certain drug medications.

Taking Alfalfa in large amounts is possibly unsafe during pregnancy and breast-feeding. Alfalfa may act like estrogen.

**I prefer Decaffeinated Tea's

Basil

Basil tea is caffeine free and very spicy in flavor and taste. Basil is known as a holy plant in India for its many health benefits

Benefits of Basil Tea:

Helps with Insomnia

Helps relieve Painful Menstruation

Is known for its Antioxidant Properties

Antiviral Properties

Antibacterial Properties

Gastro Intestinal Disorders

Nervous System Fatigue

Helps relieve Fever

Bronchitis

Renal Infections

*Basil Tea Warnings:

Use for short periods of time, up to six weeks at most. Its not known if long-term use is safe.

Black Tea

Almost 90% of all tea consumed in the West is **Black Tea**. Black tea, along with Green, White and Oolong tea are made from the leaves of the Camellia Sinensis plant, although black tea generally has more flavor and caffeine.

Benefits of Black Tea:

Abundant in antioxidants

Manganese in Black tea may reduce the risk of coronary heart disease

Promotes blood flow in the brain without over stimulating the heart

The Tannins in tea have a therapeutic effect and are a great digestive aid

Increased Energy

*Black Tea Warnings:

Drinking high amounts of Black tea containing more than 10 grams of caffeine is unsafe. High doses of Black tea can cause severe side effects.

Blessed Thistle

Blessed Thistle Herb or Blessed Tea, is native to the Mediterranean. It can be found growing in the Eastern United States and all throughout Europe. Blessed thistle has been known to increase appetite, assist digestion, stimulate saliva, stimulate gastric juice secretion and stimulate bile flow. It is also has been used as an anti-inflammatory, antioxidant, breast-stimulant and menstrual-flow stimulant.

Benefits of Blessed Thistle Tea:

Blessed Thistle tea is drunk before a meal to avoid flatulence.

Used to regulate menstruation.

Used to treat digestive problems, gout, fever, and headaches.

Can be used alone or with other herbs to aid in lactation for breastfeeding women.

Fenugreek and Blessed Milk Thistle tea helps with breast milk flow and production.

*Blessed Thistle Tea Warnings:

High amounts of Blessed Thistle tea, greater than 5 gm per cup of tea can lead to stomach irritation & vomiting.

Burdock Root

Burdock Root is used both internally as well as topically to treat many ailments and is considered to be a safe holistic treatment. Burdock produces a burr that sticks to animal fur and clothing and will cause skin irritation. Burdock grows to be approximately 2 or 3 feet tall and produces a purple flower and deep roots that are eaten as vegetable roots or used medicinally.

Benefits of Burdock Root Tea:

Reduce blood sugar levels

Decreases the amount of insulin needed in diabetics

Can be used a s a diuretic or blood cleanser

Can help treat eczema and other skin blemishes

*Burdock Root Tea Warnings:

Burdock can interact with some medications such as:

Nonsteroidal anti-inflammatory drugs

Blood thinners

Antibiotics

Catnip

Catnip is part of the mint family of herbs, and contains a substance called Nepetalactone. Nepetalactone has the same effect as a mild sedative. Catnip is popular for those suffering from insomnia.

Catnip Tea Benefits:

Antibacterial

Antifungal

Mild Sedative

Muscle Relaxant

Relieves Headaches

Relieves Stress

Reduces Pain

Used to Treat Colds

Used to Treat Bronchial Congestion

Settles an Upset Stomach

Nausea

Restlessness, nervousness

Toothache

*Catnip Tea Warnings:

Catnip may enhance the effects of alcohol

May make heavy menstrual cycles worse

May increase urination

Chamomile

Chamomile is used to treat digestive problems and aid in sleep. Chamomile can increase the potency of other plants such as mint, oregano and basil.

Benefits of Chamomile Tea:

Sleep Aid

Helps with Insomnia

Helps aid in the digestion of food

Has a calming effect on the body

*Chamomile Tea Warnings:

Chamomile may interfere with medications, increasing their sedative and cognitive effects.

Chrysanthemum

Chrysanthemum tea is infused with the sweet taste of dried chrysanthemum flowers. It is a popular spring time Chinese tea.

Chrysanthemum Tea Benefits:

Cleans the Liver

Eases Headaches and Tension

Angina

Can speed up recovery from a Cold

Helps bring down Fever

Helps in aiding Type 2 Diabetes sufferers

*Chrysanthemum Tea Warnings:

Avoid taking this tea during pregnancy, as its effects are not well known

Known to interfere with the effects of some medicines

Devils Claw

Devil's Claw gets its name from the claw shape hooks on the plant's fruit. Native to South Africa, it is primarily used medicinally with nearly all the world's supply coming from Namibia. It is primarily used to treat arthritis, back ache and tendonitis.

Devils Claw Tea Benefits:

Devil's Claw can be used externally to treat skin irritations

Reducing neck pain and inflammation due to arthritis.

Often used for internal ailments of the liver, kidneys and bladder and gall bladder.

Treatment of lower back pain

*Devils Claw Tea Warnings:

Avoid use in pregnancy

May harm people with disorders of the heart and circulatory system

Avoid mixing with prescribed medicines

May increase bile production

Avoid using devil's claw if you have gallstones

Dandelion

Dandelion Root tea is a significant source of beta-carotene, potassium, calcium, magnesium and iron. Dandelion root is used in the treatment of heartburn, chronic rheumatism, eczema, gout, diabetes and other health conditions. Dandelion aids the liver and gallbladder by removing waste material

Benefits of Dandelion Tea:

Helps with urinary tract infection

Helps to lower high levels of cholesterol

Aids in the treatment of liver disease

Increases bowel movement to stop constipation

*Dandelion Tea Warnings:

Dandelion may cause allergic reaction in people allergic to ragweed plants

Echinacea

Echinacea tea is most effect when taken before the onset of cold, sinus, gum inflammation or other infection symptoms. Echinacea is known to have a numbing sensation that relieves the pain of cold sores and also offers some protection against herpes simplex. When fighting an established virus, combining Echinacea with goldenseal or Oregon grape enhances the effectiveness. Dosage is important. You have to take enough Echinacea tea frequently to see any significant effects.

Benefits of Echinacea Tea:

Bone health

Echinacea tea includes manganese, selenium, iron, vitamin B, zinc, calcium, magnesium, and several other minerals and vitamins

Believed to have antiseptic effect

Boosts immune system

*Echinacea Tea Warnings:

Use with cautiously if you're allergic to ragweed. If you suffer from arthritis or lupus, or a chronic infection such as tuberculosis, avoid using Echinacea.

Dong Quai

Dong Quai root has been used in China, Japan and Korea for thousands of years to treat many forms of female complaints, blood ailments and stomach ailments. It is often referred to as Female Ginseng.

Dong Quai Tea Benefits:

Dong Quai is a common tea for woman as it is effective in regulating menstruation

Increases female libido.

Can be used to treat gout, athlete's foot and even acne

Helps reduce feelings of anxiety and can be used as a sedative.

Is said to be a good daily tonic for its ability to strengthen the heart and aid in all forms of stomach disorders.

*Dong Quai Tea Warnings:

Do not use if you have a cold, the flu, or diarrhea

Do not use if you are pregnant or breast-feeding

Eucalyptus

Eucalyptus tea is used to treat a variety of conditions. The Eucalyptol from the Eucalyptus tree is the source of its cooling flavor. It also contains flavonoids, quercetin, tannins and volatile oils. Many of these elements act as antioxidants. Eucalyptus tea goes well with Peppermint Tea as a mixture.

Eucalyptus Tea Benefits:

Natural Anti-Inflammatory

Lowers Blood-Sugar

Treats Nasal Congestion

Treats Bronchitis

Treats Common Cold

*Eucalyptus Tea Warnings:

Those who are pregnant or breast-feeding, have liver disease, or have intestinal tract inflammation should avoid use.

Eyebright

Eyebright tea is a tea that can benefit your eyesight. Eyebright herbs are combined with other herbs for maximum herbal benefits. Eyebright-Nettle tea is a used to fight eye irritation and viral infections.

Benefits of Eyebright Tea:

Tightens top layers of mucous membrane surrounding the eye

Reduces mucous secretions from the eyes

Creates a protective covering over the surface of the eye

Treat Eye Infections

Eyebright contains flavonoids and beta-carotene which helps to strengthen memory.

Sooth Tired Eyes

Eyebright acts as an anti-inflammatory

Relieve Nose & Sinus Irritations

Reduce Eye Fatigue

Treat Common Cold & Runny Eyes

*Eyebright Tea Warnings:

Eyebright shouldn't be used if you've had eye surgery or you wear contact lenses.

Fennel

Fennel tea and Fennel Seed tea are great holistic healers. Fennel is also used as a treatment for upper respiratory disorders, as an aid in breast milk flow and as a diuretic. It can also be used as a fever and pain reliever as well as an eye wash and appetite suppressant. Fennel acts as an excellent digestive aid to relieve abdominal cramps, gas and bloating.

Benefits of Fennel Tea:

Increases Estrogen Activity

Increases Breast Milk Flow

Reduces Pain

Antidepressant

Reduces Pain

Reduces Fever

Fennel Increases Breast Size

Eases Digestion

Lowers Blood Pressure

*Fennel Tea Warnings:

Fennel Tea may increase your skin's sensitivity to sunlight

If you have an allergy to carrots or celery avoid Fennel Tea

Ginger

Ginger tea is known to settle and upset stomach. Ginger's root contains chemicals called Gingerols and Shogaols, chemicals that relax the intestinal tract, preventing motion sickness and relieving the nausea, vomiting, colicky stomach cramps, and diarrhea that often accompany stomach flu.

Ginger Tea Benefit:

Can improve circulation

Relieves arthritic pain

Known to reduces inflammation

Relieves menstrual pain and cramping

Can improve circulation

Helps the digestive system

*Ginger Tea Warnings:

Increases the risk of bleeding in those who have bleeding disorders

Consuming ginger tea while pregnant can pose health risks

Ginkgo Biloba

Ginkgo leaf extracts are being used today to treat Alzheimer's disease, dementia and to promote memory It's leaves contain bioflavonoid, which decreases the fragility of blood capillaries and influences their permeability, increasing blood circulation in the entire body. It has been reported to be effective in treating retinal eye ailments such as macular degeneration.

Benefits of Ginkgo Biloba Tea:

Improves blood flow

Used as a memory and concentration booster

Can improve attention span

Reduces mood swings

Protects the body from free radicals

It helps reduce nerve damage

It helps reduce tinnitus

Helps with erectile dysfunction

*Ginkgo Biloba Warnings:

Excessive use of Ginkgo Biloba can thin the blood

Ginseng

Ginseng tea has been used traditionally to improve sexual performance and has been known to be an aphrodisiac for men. It comes from a family of 11 perennial plants. Ginseng gives your immune system a boost protecting against viruses and common illnesses.

Ginseng Tea Benefits:

Increases libido and sexual desire

It boosts your immune system

Is known to reduce anxiety

Reduces menstrual pain in women

Increases energy levels

Has a relaxing and soothing effect on the body

Improves signs of mental distress, asthma and arthritis

*Ginseng Tea Warnings:

A very serious allergic reaction to this product is rare

Trouble sleeping is the most common side effect

Green Tea

Green tea enhances overall health and can help fight against serious complications and health issues, particularly cardiovascular conditions. Consumption of Green tea leads to improved learning ability and memory. Green tea provides the body vital antioxidants and prevents immature aging.

Green Tea Benefits:

Reduces Cholesterol

Antioxidants in Green tea are beneficial for the skin

Managing Diabetes

Can help prevent and reduce the risk of rheumatoid arthritis

Helps relieve stress and anxiety

Boosts the immune system

Honeysuckle

Honeysuckle flowers are known for eliminating toxins from the body and for breaking up cold and fever. It also used as a detoxifier, eliminating all unwanted toxins from the body safely, as opposed to using an over the counter detox medicine. Honeysuckle contains calcium, magnesium, potassium, vitamin C, and Rutin, a nutrient that enhances the effectiveness of vitamin C.

Honeysuckle Tea Benefits:

Can help improve respiratory illness

Can help in dealing with headaches

Eases sore joints and reduce inflammation

Inhibits the bacteria that causes salmonella, strep, staph and tuberculosis infections

*Honeysuckle Tea Warnings:

Skin contact with honeysuckle can cause rash in allergic people

Hops

Hops tea has traditionally been used to relieve tension, stress, anxiety and helps people who deal with bouts of insomnia. Hops is widely known as a powerful natural sedative which can help with sleepless, restless nights with no side effects. Hops are often blended with the following herbs: Passion Flower, Valerian and Chamomile.

Hops Tea Benefits:

Used to improve appetite

Used to prevent indigestion

Helps aid in dealing with pain from menstrual cramps

Can help increase the flow of urine

Used as a bitter herb tonic

*Hops Tea Warnings:

Hops may make depression worse

Hyssop

Hyssop is said to mean Holy Herb. Hyssop tea has been used as an expectorant which clears mucus from the throat and lungs, as well as an anti-inflammatory aid.

Hyssop Tea Benefits:

Hyssop tea is often used for chest congestion and cases of bronchitis.

Used as an antiviral agent

Relieves tension, gas and abdominal pain such as cramping

*Hyssop Warning:

Hyssop shouldn't be used during pregnancy.

Hyssop has been associated with causing seizures when used excessively

Hyssop contains iodine and shouldn't be used by people suffering from hyperthyroid disorders.

Jasmine

Jasmine tea has been found to eliminate harmful bacteria and ease chronic inflammation. If you suffer from cardiovascular issues, Jasmine tea can help in preventing further problems.

Benefits of Jasmine Tea:

It relieves stress

Provides a calming and soothing effect

Relieves tension from headaches, aching muscles and anxiety

May help in preventing cancer

Can reverse the negative effects of diabetes

Strengthens the immune system

Increases your metabolism

Antibacterial

High in Antioxidants

Peppermint

Peppermint tea is widely known for its ability to lessen the pain associated with sinus problems and headaches. Peppermint tea stops headache pain by opening up the brain's constricted blood vessels. It is also a popular tea for treating an upset stomach.

Peppermint Tea Benefits:

Treats Menstrual Cramps

Its fresh flavor can prevent bad breath

Is used to strengthen the immune system

*Peppermint Tea Warnings

If you suffer from acid reflux disease, it is best to avoid Peppermint tea or Peppermints of any kind. It relaxes the sphincter muscle of the stomach and esophagus causing more of a chance for the acid to flow from the stomach to the throat and cause heart burn.

Valerian Root

Valerian root has been widely praised for its sedative properties. It is used in aiding those dealing with bouts of insomnia as well as calming the body in times of pain. Unlike most sleep or pain medications, Valerian root, when taken in moderate doses is a potent herb without the terrible side effects.

Valerian Root Benefits:

Powerful sedative without the major side effects found in sleep medications

Used to treat nervous anxiety

Non addictive, Non habit forming

Known as a muscle relaxer that can aid in the pain associated with cramps

Helps in the cessation of smoking and nicotine addiction

*Valerian Root Warnings:

Doctors warn against taking Valerian Root when taking any other sedative

Taking Valerian Root for too long may cause an Inability to sleep

THE END

Be sure to check out my other publications:

-Fly Ty's Book of Poems

-Fly Ty's Book of Poetry volume 2

-Intimate Thoughts of an Original Man

(Fly Ty's Book of Poetry Volume 3)

-Destiny's First Day –

A look at African American Hair Issues (Short Story)

(Written By: Fly Ty Unchained)

-A Message to Our Suns -

(Listen up Young Man)

(Written By: Fly Ty Unchained)

-Fly Ty Unchained Presents:

(Letters from the Diaspora)

(Written By: Fly Ty Unchained and Various

Writers, Poets and Spoken Word Artists)

-Locs, Life and Love Pt 1 The Knotty Chroniclez

(Written By: Andre'a Deberry & Fly Ty Unchained)

-Locs, Life and Love Pt 2 The Knotty Chroniclez

(Written By: Andre'a Deberry & Fly Ty Unchained)

-Scatter Brain!-

(Written By: Fly Ty Unchained)

-Just Speak Your Mind -

(Written By: Fly Ty Unchained, Various Poets, Writers)

-E.McCiers Tasteful Thoughts -

(Featuring Fly Ty's Fruit Smoothies and Juices)

(Written By: Fly Ty Unchained, Erica McCier)

-Fly Ty's Famous Fruit Smoothies and Juice Recipes

(Written By Fly Ty Unchained)

-Money Is The New Father -

(Written By: Fly Ty Unchained)

-Friends With Benefits-

(Written By: Fly Ty Unchained & Erica McCier)

-Just Speak Your Mind Pt 2-

(Written By: Fly Ty Unchained and Various Writers)

-The Knotty Dread Diaries - DKJ Edition (Hardcover)

(Written By: Fly Ty Unchained and Various Writers)

-Life of a Single Father-

(Written By: Fly Ty Unchained)

-He Said / She Said-

(Written By: Fly Ty Unchained, Lisa Michelle)

-The ILLUMI-KNOTTY Diaries-

(Written By: Fly Ty Unchained and The ILLUMI-KNOTTY)

All available on:

Lulu.com/spotlight/FlyboyTy

You can also contact me at:

madeintheimageofgod@yahoo.com

FLY TY UNCHAINED 2015